Always Unstable

Bipolar and Hospitalisation. A Memoir.
By Meghan Shultz

For Travis, Mum, and Dad,
Thanks for putting up with me.
Thanks for not walking away.

Forward

It was always there really. Ever since I was a child. I'll be the first to say that I was kind of strange when I was a kid. When I was in kindergarten I had this weird thing about toilets where I would only use the toilet that had no door. I was afraid to be shut in the cubicle. I hated being separated from my Mum too. I would scream and cry so much, the teacher would have to hold me back just so that my Mum could leave. I didn't like being around people. I had more invisible friends than actual friends. I was always nervous and anxious. I was terrified of the dark because I was afraid of the things that I saw and heard in it. I started hallucinating at a very young age.

It wasn't until I was around 10 or 11 years old that I started to realize just how fucking miserable I was. But I thought that it was normal. That is when I started to fantasize about suicide. It just got worse and worse and by the time I reached high school at age 13, I was already starting to hurt myself. At first I was ashamed and I didn't want anyone to see what I was doing to myself but it escalated pretty quickly.

I found self- harm to be a calming release. I could exhale, I could feel something. Emotionally I felt nothing, I felt numb. Cutting helped me to feel something physically painful to try and make up for that. It was a wonderful release. Given, not the best way to express my pain, I don't recommend it, but at the time I didn't know how else to express the pain that I was experiencing.

I had no idea what was going on inside of my head. I didn't know that I had a Mental Illness, I didn't know that I was sick. I knew that there was something wrong with me, but I didn't know that I was sick. I didn't know that it was okay to be sick, that it was an illness and I need not be ashamed of it. My family didn't know. I never told anyone. I felt so much shame and confusion, fear, pain. I just couldn't figure it out. What was wrong with me?

I've been mentally ill for basically my whole life. I have Bipolar I Disorder, Borderline Personality Disorder, and Anxiety Disorder. I honestly don't know what it's like to live without a mental illness. I don't know what it's like to be without euphoric highs and devastating lows. Being mentally ill can be terrifying. Mental illness can seem like an unstoppable force at times. For me, it's a constant back and forth between Mania, Depression, Psychosis, and Mixed Episodes. Around and around and around. Unrelenting. Suffocating. It makes me want to scream and cry out in pain, even though I really can't feel anything at all.

Let's start with Mania.

Mania, for the most part, is horrible. It can have its upsides, sure, but mostly I find it to be horrible. Sometimes it's like being full of some divine energy, a strong, unrelenting, euphoric energy. The energy is filling me and I feel like I might explode and my mind is going at a million miles an hour. There are far too many things in my head for me to process. I talk a lot and I talk over people, I don't let them get a word in edge ways. My words trip over each other when I talk, I can't get them out quick enough. I race around, cleaning my apartment, I can't sit still, I'm always fidgeting. I never want to sleep and when I try to sleep I still can't stop moving. I just lay there, fidgeting.

On the outset mania can seem incredibly appealing. Hell, when I'm in a depressive episode all I wish for is mania. Mania can be fun and exciting. It can be thrilling. There was this one time where I bought myself loads and loads of balloons. I wanted to fill my closet with them so that I could have dance parties in there. And that's exactly what I did. I blew them all up by mouth too. I had my very own balloon room. And I danced in it frequently.

Mania often gives me a confidence that I never thought I had. I don't know where it came from but hey, it's there! It makes me a different person, a person that I think I am, that I think I want to be. I've been promoted at work multiple times while manic, I just volunteer myself for everything, I work hard at everything. And I kick ass at it.

Then there's all of the hobbies. I go through hobbies like a chain smoker goes through cigarettes; to the next, to the next. Piano, Saxophone, Stamp collecting, Coin collecting, Violin, French, German, Sign Language, Knitting, Colouring. Some of the hobbies don't even last long enough for me to get the stuff in the mail. Like sign language, I was over that one before I even got the books in the mail. There's also religion, I once became obsessed with Catholicism and another time, Buddhism, then Wicca. I also like to shop and there's usually a theme. Sometimes I will buy a lot of sweaters, sometimes I'm into makeup, even though I rarely wear make-up. Often, I'm into stationery and books. I buy so many books yet lack the required concentration to actually read them all. Needless to say, I have quite a large credit card debt. I not only maxed out my own credit cards but also my husband's.

Mania can be so thrilling and so much fun. But it's also devastating and destroying. It's a rollercoaster ride, from hell. It can be terrifying. Throwing me one way and then the other. You're left with a whole lot of mess, debt, picking up the pieces can be tough. Mania can also put a lot of strain on relationships. When I'm manic I never spare a thought for anyone else, I don't care who I hurt. Just so long as I'm having fun and doing what I like.

Mania isn't always an up kind of mood either. Sometimes it is extreme and unrelenting anger. Irritability, moodiness, I snap at everyone for no reason. I hate everyone. I don't want to be near anyone because I'm so angry for no reason. This is also mania. I asked my Husband once how he puts up with it, he replied and said that it's a lot like Stockholm Syndrome.

Then there's Depression.

Depression consumes me. It grabs me, holds me, and never lets me go. It suffocates me, I can't breathe, I struggle against it. After a while I just stop fighting it. Because what's the point? No one likes me. No one loves me. Everybody hates me. That's not true, but that's how it feels. I have so much contempt and disgust for myself that I can't see how anybody else could possibly like me or love me.

I can't get out of bed, but I don't ever sleep. I just lay there and stare at the wall. Never quite finding the will to move because I'm still trying to think of a reason to live. When I do get up......well it's no different except that I'm sitting somewhere else, staring at a different wall. I want to be alone but at the same time, being alone is so dangerous. I can't trust myself not to hurt myself. I entertain so many thoughts of suicide, I can't guarantee that I won't attempt it. The thoughts are always there. Always terrorizing me. Haunting me. Pulling me down.

Depression is unrelenting. I wish and hope for mania, even though that's just as dangerous. I sit and sit and just wait for my mood to flip.

Then there's my old friend Psychosis...

Psychosis happens in both manic and depressive episodes for me. I have auditory and visual hallucinations on a regular basis. Even though I'm on medication they're still not 100% gone. I also have delusions, mostly of the paranoid kind. Delusional thinking can be especially difficult. There was once when I wouldn't trust my pharmacy with my medications. I thought that they were trying to poison me by coating my medications in an invisible layer of poison every time they filled my prescriptions. I was stable enough to know that I had to take my medications but it was still incredibly difficult to get past those thoughts.

Mixed episodes.......they're just pure hell. It's like mania and depression mixed together and it's absolutely horrific. A lot of anger, a lot of energy, and a lot of suicidal and destructive thoughts.

I've been through almost 30 different medications in different combinations plus Electroconvulsive Therapy. Nothing ever works and if it does it's not for very long.

I'm so tired. Tired of what is, of what's to come. It is a disease that exhausts and never leaves. I have all of the energy in the world when I'm manic but once I crash, I feel it. I feel every ache in my bones, I feel the hurricane in my mind, going and going and going. Never stopping. Not for a minute.

I've been hospitalized five times. Once as a teenager and then four more times all within one year as an adult. These are the stories of each of those hospitalizations. What triggered them and took me there, what happened while I was there, and what happened afterwards.

I'm telling it like it is. Some of it may be graphic and triggering. Please beware.

Hospital V.1
The Suicide Attempt

1.1

I walked into my room, dropping my school bag onto the floor and kicking off my shoes as I went. The late afternoon sun was still shining through my window. I jumped up on to my bed to reach the blind and pulled it down roughly. I hate the sun, it's so bright and imposing. Miserable, shitting thing.

I fell down onto my bed and gathered up the covers around me as I leaned up against my bed frame. I turned on the radio and let my mind wander for a short while before bringing myself back to reality. Today is a special day. Today is the day that I am going to die. I will never wake up again, I've already seen my last sunrise and for some reason that filled me with an unbelievable sense of calm. I didn't have to do this anymore. No more hurting, no more pain. No more voices and noise in my head. I will never wake up again. Everything is going to stop.

I looked around my room at all of my possession's and briefly wondered what they'll do with them. Will they keep them all, just as they are? Or will it cause too much pain, will they throw them all away? I looked down next to me at Jemima

Puddle Duck. Someone gave her to me when I was born, I've slept with her almost every night of my life. I must make sure to leave a note that she be buried or cremated with me.

My left wrist started to ache. I rolled up my sleeve and took off my watch and the band aids. I used to cut myself just enough that I could fit it under my watch. But it was everywhere over my forearm now. I could never hope to cover it merely with a watch again. It now required constant long sleeves and band aids. I picked at one of the fresh wounds until it started to slowly seep blood again. It wasn't enough though, I needed more. I leant under my bed to find my blade. There was something about cutting that I found calming. The feel of the blade, the feel of the blood seeping out. It was my go to coping mechanism. As I cut I could feel my heart rate slowing, my body relaxing. I laid back and closed my eyes. I wouldn't have to do this for much longer, I thought to myself. But I would miss it.

Just one more thing to do before I go. Today is piano lesson day. I loved the piano, I truly did. I'd been having lessons for about four of five years now. But I wasn't the best. I couldn't do something that I wasn't the best at. But one more

11

lesson couldn't hurt. Mum was already waiting in the car so I pulled down my sleeve, grabbed my books and ran outside to meet her. My Brother and Sister came too. My lessons were only half an hour long and afterwards we would always get dinner from the chicken shop across the street.

My piano lesson felt like it went on forever. I was so eager to get home. Eager but nervous at the same time. I waited in the kitchen for my serving of dinner and then took it with me to my room. I sat it on my bed and waited in my room for everyone else to leave the kitchen. All of the pills were kept in the kitchen and I didn't want anybody to see what I was doing.

I walked down the dark hall and into the kitchen. The pills were in the pantry. I walked over and turned the pantry light on. I took every pill that I could find in there, every box, every bottle. I took them back to my room.

I threw them all on my bed next to where my dinner was sitting. It might be worth mentioning at this point, but I couldn't swallow pills. Every time I had a headache or needed an antibiotic I had to have a liquid medicine. I had never been able to swallow tablets, not like now. Now I can swallow a fist full at a time, at one point I was on twenty pills a day. The problem back then was that I always felt like they got stuck in my throat. But that night I was determined, and I had a plan.

I took the pills, one at a time. After every pill I had to have a bite of food. That was my plan. One pill, one bite of food. Pill, food, pill, food. It's a good thing that I had a lot of dinner because I had a lot of pills. So on I went, pill then food, pill then food. It took a long time to get the pills down. But I did it. I was so proud of myself.

When I was done I got into bed and turned on the radio. Music. I wanted to listen to music as I went. The rest of the plan was that I would gently drift off to sleep and never wake up again. A fool proof plan, so I thought.

1.2

I slowly opened my eyes. My head was aching; my mouth was dry. I felt like I was going to be sick. And that's when I realized.... I'm still alive. I stopped still for the briefest of seconds, heart racing, breathing heavy and then...

WHAT

THE

FUCK!!!

I screamed into my pillow, crying, starting to hyperventilate. Why the fuck is this happening?! Why am I being punished?! I sat up, holding my head in my hands grabbing at fistfuls of my hair. I took so many pills. So many. This shouldn't be happening. Someone should be finding my cold, lifeless body right now. The pain was overwhelming. Not the physical pain, the emotional pain. Although the pain in my stomach was starting to become more aggressive. I leaned over the side of my bed and grabbed my trash can just in time. I lay over the edge of my bed for a while, waiting to throw up again.

It was a school day, my Mum had been knocking on my bedroom door in an effort to get me out of bed. I pulled myself up and walked over to my bedroom door. I hesitated for a moment before opening it and walking out across the hall, into the living room. My Mum was sitting in her usual spot, on the rocking chair next to the heater.

"Mum? I'm not going to school today. I don't feel well." I spat out as quick as I could before turning around and going back to my bedroom. I grabbed my trash can as I felt myself heave again. I climbed back into my bed and under my covers. Warm and comforting at least. I thought that maybe if I could only get back to sleep, I might still have a chance to die. Maybe I wouldn't be so unlucky as to wake up a second time. Close your eyes Meghan, just close your eyes. You can do this, you can die.

I woke up again. It was dark outside now. I was in so much pain, clutching my stomach as it churned and burned. I had to tell someone. I sat up on the edge of my bed, scared. How do you tell your Mum that you did something so horrible? How do you tell a parent you don't want the life that they have given you? I guess there is no good way.

"Mum, I think I need to go to the hospital to get my stomach pumped". I stood frozen.

"What?" She said.

"I took too many pills. But I took them yesterday and I'm still alive and I feel really sick and I don't want to feel sick anymore so I think that I should get my stomach pumped."

She stood there in shock. I wanted so bad for her to say something, anything. Becoming animated again, she picked up the phone and looked at me, "How many did you take? What did you take?"

"I dunno, everything that I could find......."

She got off the phone with the poisons information line, looked up and told me to get in the car. She was going to drive me to the hospital in the city. I guess it had been long enough since the overdose, it was unlikely that I was going to die if I hadn't already. That really wasn't comforting.

I was afraid. I hadn't ever counted on having to face what I did, to see the pain on my mother's face. I never wanted to hurt anyone, it never occurred to me that I would to be honest. I was convinced that no one would even miss me.

When we got to the hospital we were seated briefly in the waiting area. I didn't have to wait very long for a bed. The doctors asked me a lot of questions about what I took and how much. They had me hooked up to a drip. I don't know what was in it. While they were examining me they pulled up the sleeves of my sweater. My left arm, there were cuts everywhere. Some of them deep, some of them artificial. My Mum was sitting right there when they did this, she didn't know about the self-harm before that moment. I had it hidden so well, nobody knew about it. I was so ashamed. I had never really been ashamed of it until this moment. The hurt that I had caused. Still to this day I can't think about that moment without tearing up. I never wanted to hurt anyone, I never thought that I would.

Eventually, I was moved up stairs to an adolescent ward for the night. So they could watch me and make sure that, physically, I was going to be okay. And I was, physically okay. Mentally I was a fucking train wreck.

1.3

The next day when I came off of the drip, I was moved to another unit. I was moved to the adolescent psychiatric unit. It was terrifying. It never occurred to me before this point, just how messed up I really was. But oh boy, did it occur to me now. It had been escalating for years. And now, here, I understood that maybe I was legitimately insane. Terrifying although it was, maybe it was also relieving, maybe this meant that there was a possibility of recovery, change, healing. I guess time will tell.

They roomed me right across from the nurse's station. I was on suicide watch. I had a single room and bathroom, I was constantly checked on, I couldn't have my doors closed all of the way, I wasn't allowed to shave my legs.

Yet they didn't medicate me. Nope. To this day I never understood why. It seemed as if every other patient was being medicated except for me. It's not that I wanted to take medication, I really didn't, but I had just tried to kill myself. Was I not depressed enough for them? That aside, I was diagnosed at the time with 'Psychotic Depression'. Apparently the things that were in my head were just that, in my head, not real. I had been having hallucinations and delusions on top of having depression. I thought that I was talking to dead people. I was having full on conversations with people that weren't really there, I was hallucinating evil dolls. But I thought that they were real. Before then it never even occurred to me that they were hallucinations.

After a few days I had settled into somewhat of a routine. It consisted of laying on my bed, crying and avoiding all people. I would get up for lunch though. I had spaghetti and meatballs every day for lunch for the time that I was there because it seemed like the only edible food. For dinner I ate fish and chips. I would eat it at the table near the nurses' station then go back to my room and hide away. Despite my apparent unsocial-ness however, I did make a couple of friends. They were also there for attempted suicide. We could relate to each other.

After four or five days I was moved into a room called 'The Bay'. There was a bunch of us all roomed together in there, maybe 6 or 7 of us. I hated it instantly. I hated to be around so many people. I've never really liked to be near people. It was too much. I huddled into the corner next to my bed which was in the far corner of the room. It wasn't bed time so I was the only one in there. I needed to hurt myself, I needed to feel pain, cause pain. It's amazing how easily I feel self-destructive again. So I sat there, and I dug into the skin of my ankle with my thumb nail. I dug and scratched away at it until it started to bleed. Eventually, a nurse came to see what I was up to. She saw what I was doing to myself and had me moved to another room. A room where I only had one roommate. To this day, I always grow my nails when I'm in hospital, just in case I need to hurt myself.

1.4

I was in hospital for nearly two weeks, from memory. About half way through my stay though they allowed me to leave for an overnight stay with my Aunt and Uncle. I was excited but scared at the same time. Excited to get out for a bit but scared that I might hurt myself. I didn't hurt myself though. We went shopping in a nearby mall. My Aunt bought me some new clothes which included a jacket that I still have to this day. It's a damn comfy jacket. I stayed overnight and then went back to the hospital the next day.

After about a week and a half my parents were called in for a meeting with the team that was treating me. Basically to tell them what was wrong with me, Psychotic Depression and Anxiety. Shortly after that I was discharged. I was not fixed, I was not better, I was not well. But I still didn't feel sick enough to really ask for more help. I still felt ashamed of myself. I took the fact that they didn't medicate me as a sign that I wasn't really sick. So I went home, unmedicated, still hallucinating, still delusional, still hearing voices, still suicidal, and still thinking that I wasn't sick enough for anyone to bother helping me. You would think that after leaving hospital, things would start to get better. But no, they just kept getting worse.

I was matched up with a psychologist. I saw her about once a week/ once every couple of weeks. I didn't really like her a great deal. I have a thing about female doctors and psychologists, I just don't like them. I don't know why; I just feel more comfortable around male health professionals. Having said that, there have been some female doctors over the years that I have really loved, just not many.

Eventually, maybe about six months or so after I left the hospital, they did start medicating me. I was clearly no better and still hurting myself so they had to do something. My doctor had started giving me antidepressants. I wasn't responding well to them though. The problem was that the antidepressants would make me so high, and then I would crash and burn. I would go back and tell him that they weren't working when what was actually happening was the antidepressants were causing mania and then I would crash back into depression. My doctor never knew this because I never told him. I thought that the mania was normal happiness. I thought that it was how every normal person felt. He tried a few different ones before ordering me a consult with the visiting Psychiatrist. He saw me once and then diagnosed me with Schizoaffective Disorder Depressive type. I didn't really know anything about it. I knew that I was depressed, I knew that I was 'psychotic'. I guess that's all that really mattered. I knew what was wrong now, so how do I fix it?

1.5

After seeing the Psychiatrist, I was immediately put on an antipsychotic. It made me sleepy. So sleepy. What to do with something that makes you sleep? Take half the box and see how long I can sleep for. I slept for nearly two days. I stopped taking them after that. Yeah, they helped with the psychotic symptoms but I was still depressed as shit. Besides, my doctor found out what I did and started limiting me to a week's supply at a time. I felt insulted that he didn't trust me with them, even though he did the right thing. I really couldn't be trusted with my medication.

It didn't take long before I moved onto something much more thrilling, illicit drugs, alcohol, and cigarettes. I started smoking pot and smoking cigarettes shortly before turning 16. I also started causing trouble at school and getting detention all of the time. I just didn't want to be there. Sometimes I didn't even bother to show up to school at all. I would forge notes from my mum so that they wouldn't write home asking where I was. When I finally did turn 16 I stopped going to school completely. I am a high school dropout. I had been working but I also walked out of my job shortly after I dropped out of school. Literally, walked out half way through helping a customer because I started crying out of nowhere and it wouldn't stop. I was a mess.

After I left school I started to get into drugs a lot more, I also started to drink a lot. This went on for a few years. I would take just about anything that I could get my hands on, Marijuana, LSD, Magic Mushrooms, Meth, Speed, Ecstasy…. the list goes on. I was just drinking and drugging myself into oblivion. I was miserable, I was a mess. But at least I could feel something different, right? I thought that the drugs were helping me but really they were all just making things so much worse.

I was working on and off during this time before landing a permanent job in my late teens. While I wasn't working I would sometimes steal money from my Mums bill money to help pay for my drug and alcohol habit. I would then lie when she asked me about it. Of every single horrible, miserable thing that I have done (and there's a lot), this is the thing that I feel the guiltiest about it, lying and stealing from my mother.

Through this time my biggest problem was the drinking. Yes, drugs are probably worse but my biggest problem was drinking. I would drink almost every night of the week. I smoked meth so that I could tolerate my alcohol and drink more. I rarely slept at night, I would sleep during the day instead. I was often so hungover during the day though that I probably couldn't get up if I tried anyway.

In my early twenties, after a long term relationship ended I started to go clubbing in the city a lot and eventually got a transfer with work so that I could move to the city. Clubbing meant a lot of alcohol, ecstasy, and meth. I had boyfriends during this time but I always cheated. I was basically just slutting it up for a while there. I remember one morning in particular, waking up, incredibly hungover, in someone's bed, about an hour out of the city. I didn't care who I hurt. I wanted what I wanted and I wanted it now. I was like a tornado. I was destructive, to myself and to other people. It was to the point where my own sister wouldn't even speak to me anymore. But I didn't care. This went on for about a year or so. Eventually though, I did get through it.

Hospital V.2
The Mixed Episode

2.1

In 2010 my husband and I started dating. We were dating via the internet. We'd never met before, not in real life. We met on the internet a few years back via a website for a band that we both liked. I'm Australian and was living in Australia and he is American and was living in the grand old US of A. We met for the first time in person in January of 2011.

As soon as we met each other in person we decided that we wanted to get married so when I got back from America I lodged my visa application straight away. The wait was HORRIBLE, it took around 6 or 7 months for my application to get approved. While we were waiting we talked to each other constantly through the day via Facebook and we skyped every single night. It was honestly exhausting. In October of 2011 I finally moved. We were married a month later in November. We had just a small wedding with a handful of people. We didn't need any kind of huge event. It wasn't our style. We had our reception at an IHOP because I wanted something American. We bought our own cake. We've been married ever since. I still don't understand why he puts up with my shit though. I guess I'm just lucky.

My husband has been a really good influence on me. He is a big part of the reason why I no longer drink, smoke, or take illicit drugs. I say in part because I also had to really want to quit, I couldn't have done it if I didn't really want to. And it didn't happen all at once. First went the drugs, then the alcohol and then the cigarettes. Actually, the cigarettes went a couple of times, from memory I think that I had to quit those three or four times. I really loved smoking. I still miss it.

Anyway, I was in a new country, newly married, and living a new life of being clean. I had been clean for about a year but I know that it is something that I will always struggle with. I will always be an addict. To this day I still can't be around drugs and alcohol. The first few months in the US I did struggle a bit with depression before coming good for a while. When the depression started to get bad again I couldn't afford to see a doctor so I enrolled in a drug trial for an antidepressant. It made me manic and then I crashed. Still, I did not know that it was mania so I didn't think to mention it to anyone. Even though

I did have some problems with depression and mania, the first couple of years that I was in the US were pretty uneventful. And it was nice. For the first time in my life I didn't feel completely horrible. I was depressed but not suicidal and I wasn't self-harming. But of course, that couldn't last forever. The thing about Bipolar Disorder is that it doesn't just go away. It's not curable. It's there forever.

2.2

When I was allowed to start working in the US I got a job at a huge grocery chain. Again, I wanted something American. I loved my job. I started in the jewelry department and also worked as a cashier and in the bakery department before being promoted to a Department Manager. Doesn't sound very interesting but I loved it. I was just plodding a long, doing my thing. Then one day I decided that I wanted to get promoted again. I walked into my boss's office and asked her about being promoted to the next level of supervisor up. There was a position about to open up so she told me to go on and apply for it. It wasn't long before I was interviewed and offered the position. I was thrilled. I was going to kick ass at this job. And I did. Until I didn't.

I worked my ass off. It was coming up to inventory and I was offered basically unlimited over time. I was working 12+ hours a day, 6 days a week. Anyone can do that right? I was also only sleeping a couple of hours a night, if that. This went on for about two months if I recall correctly. I was manic. So fucking manic. Until one day when it stopped. The crash was brutal.

I was crying. I swear I woke up already crying. Not small crying either, I'm talking big ugly crying. I couldn't breathe, I felt like I was suffocating and drowning in tears. I went into the living room so that I didn't wake up my husband, he was working night shift so he slept during the day time. I was suicidal and laying on the living room floor in a ball, crying. I feared for my life, what I would do to myself, I knew what I was capable of. I decided to go find a doctor.

It was a Sunday afternoon and summer in Arizona. The nearest doctors clinic that was open was about 3 miles away. I didn't want to wake my husband and I also didn't want him to see me like this. So I walked, 3 miles in 115F heat. I wore my sunglasses so that no one could see my tears. I guess it was lucky that it was so hot and sunny outside so the sunglasses didn't look at all out of place. Maybe I could even pass off my tears as sweat.

When I got to the clinic I was dripping with sweat from the walk and still crying. It just wouldn't stop. Thankfully there was only one other person in front of me. I left my sunglasses on while I waited. The sweat was so gross; I was sticking to the plastic chair that I was sitting on.

I didn't have to wait very long before my name was called. They weighed me etc and then made me piss in a cup. They were testing me for drugs. I probably did look like an addict, I was pretty messy. I was still crying. I guess I couldn't blame them. They asked me to sit down in the doctors office and wait for her. I didn't have to wait for very long. She came in, sat down, and asked what she could do for me. I told her that I was depressed and couldn't stop crying, literally could not stop. She asked me how and when it started and I said today but I also told her my history of mental illness and depression.

She prescribed me an antidepressant before letting me go. She diagnosed me with depression and anxiety. Surprise, surprise, like I haven't been here before. I took my prescription to the nearest pharmacy and got it filled before walking back home. By now I had managed to stop crying. Now I had the hope of the antidepressant helping me.

I started taking the pills straight away. It had been a while since I'd had antidepressants, two years I think. I hadn't had this one before so I wasn't quite sure what to expect from it. Would I get happy and crash again? I hope not.

I woke up the next morning feeling like I was going to throw up. I grabbed my stomach and raced into the bathroom to lean over the toilet. Nothing. I got up and started getting ready for work. My husband was going to drive me to work, he didn't know about my trip to the doctors yet. I got into the car, still feeling ill. I turned to look at him and told him about where I went yesterday. At first he was hurt that I hadn't already told him or that I hadn't asked him to take me to the clinic the day before. He asked if I wanted to call in sick from work but I couldn't, I hated calling in sick. That would be like admitting that it's really that bad.

I should have just stayed home. I lasted about 45 minutes at work before I called my husband and asked him to come back and pick me up. I felt so sick but at the same time, something was happening. I felt as light as air, I felt like I could fly. I had so much energy, my head was racing, going a million miles an hour. I was manic. REALLY manic. Again. But I didn't know. I thought that I had depression, the doctors always say that it's depression. I was so confused; I didn't know what was happening. So I made an appointment to see another doctor.

2.3

Sitting in the waiting room waiting to see my new doctor, I was nervous. I didn't know what to expect. I still couldn't sit still it had been a week since I started the antidepressant. I was exhausted but I just couldn't stop. His assistant called my name, I got up and followed her into the doctor's office. I tried to sit still as she took my blood pressure and temperature but I just couldn't and she soon gave up on it. She told me to sit and wait, the doctor would be in shortly.

I couldn't stop fidgeting. I had restless legs, I was moving my hands around, picking at my nails and skin. The doctor came in. I looked up. He greeted me, he was very, very friendly. He took some time to ask me why I was there and what I needed. I told him about the antidepressant and my history with psychiatric problems and medications. I told him about my past substance abuse but that I was clean now and had been for a number of years. I told him that I have depression and anxiety. He said no.

"You have Bipolar Disorder. Antidepressants make you manic. Now I'm going to give you a prescription for a mood stabilizer to take with the antidepressant. You will also need to make an appointment with a Psychiatrist and find yourself a Therapist. Do you know what Bipolar Disorder is?" he asked me. "I'll have the receptionist print you out an information sheet."

I'd heard about it. I'd read about it briefly before on the internet before. I just nodded my head. I didn't know what to say. I had nothing to say, nothing but thank you and goodbye. I got my prescription, paid my co pay and left. I was in a state of shock.

I sat in silence as my husband and I left the doctors clinic and went to the pharmacy to fill my prescription. My husband asked about my appointment but I didn't know what to say. My head was so full of everything. Not only did I have all of my racing thoughts and energy to contend with, I now had a new diagnosis which I really didn't know a whole lot about. I felt so lost. Confused. Did I really have Bipolar Disorder? I tried so hard to see it but I just couldn't grasp it. It scared me.

I started taking the mood stabiliser straight away. I also found myself a Psychiatrist and a Psychologist. I had appointments set up with both of them within the coming weeks. Until then, I didn't know what to do. I just tried to go about my business as usual.

After about a week I started to notice the mood stabilizer working. I was calming down, my mood becoming more even. I felt like I could breathe again; I could sleep too. I met with my new Psychiatrist, he was very friendly, calming, patient, kind, but obviously very serious about his job. He was also kind of good looking; I have to say. He changed my meds a little and then sent me on my way with an appointment to come back the following week. I felt a small amount of hope. I was feeling better. So maybe this was manageable. Maybe Bipolar isn't so scary after all.

I met my new Therapist that week also. He was very nice. Patient also, just like my Psychiatrist. I choose doctors well it seems. I didn't talk much though. I mostly just sat there and cried. But it felt good. I was also quite stand-offish. I always have been in therapy. I want to talk but at the same time......I really don't. It's uncomfortable. I don't know why. I want to empty everything that's in my head but I'm also so scared of being judged. There's some pretty fucked up stuff in my head. So I wrote an essay. I gave it to him at my next appointment. When he was done reading it I kept the essay. I decided that I should keep it to give to future therapists. It was 6 pages long. I don't want to keep rewriting the same essay forever, 3 or 4 times is enough.

So it went on like this for a few months, medication changes and adjustments, going to therapy every Monday morning and crying. But then, it all just fell apart. I don't know why, I don't know how, it just did. I wasn't just crying in the safety of my own apartment, I was also crying every day at work. One day one of my bosses noticed my crying as she walked by. She stopped to ask me what was wrong.

"Just ignore it, it happens all of the time, I'm used to it", I said

"You shouldn't have to be used to that", She replied as she walked away.

I knew she was right but what could I do?

I had an appointment with my Psychiatrist coming up, I decided that I would bring it up with him. I hadn't told him about my crying yet, I was so ashamed of it. I was ashamed because there was no reason for it. I couldn't find one. But it just kept coming. Day after day after day. And I didn't want to live anymore. I was so tired of fighting and trying and getting nowhere. Every time things started to get better they quickly went to shit again. My psychiatrist was working so hard to find me the right medications but still, nothing was working. We'd completely ruled out any and all antidepressants, it was very clear that they weren't good for me. I don't know what he's going to try next. What else is there?

2.4

Today was Psychiatrist day. I was scared and nervous. Afraid about what I had to tell him and of what he would say.

"Doctor……", I hesitated while fidgeting in my chair, "There's something that I need to tell you. I can't stop crying. Every day, I just cry and cry and cry. I don't even know why I'm crying. It just keeps coming. I'm tired, I don't want to do this anymore, I can't", I pleaded.

He asked me, calmly, "Are you suicidal, are you going to hurt yourself?"

"Yes. I want to find a really tall building, I want to stand on the ledge, backwards. I want to fall off of the building backwards so that I can feel like I'm flying, feel like I'm free, right before I die". I couldn't look at him while I spoke. I was so ashamed of what I had said. But it was true, that's what I wanted to do.

He thought for just a moment. "You need to go to the hospital today. Here is their information, their address. Can your husband take you there?" He handed me a sheet with all of the hospitals information, phone number etc.

I sat there, stunned. I hadn't been in a psychiatric hospital since I was 15. It never even crossed my mind to go. But there I sat, faced with the decision. Will I or won't I. I couldn't go. I couldn't. What about work? What would I tell my family? I begged and I pleaded. I promised that I wouldn't hurt myself. Eventually he struck me a deal. He wouldn't force me to go that day on the condition that I come back next week with my husband so that he could talk with him as well. And so I left.

I didn't last two days after seeing my Psychiatrist. I called him to let him know that I was going to go to the hospital that night, and to cancel my appointment. My husband got home from work at around 9pm. I already had my things packed and I was ready to go. We stopped at the store on the way so I could get some shampoo and things, I had already been on the website to see what I could and could not bring with me. It was a dual diagnosis hospital so nothing with alcohol within the first four ingredients. Hence the need for new shampoo and things.

We got to the hospital and I had no idea what to expect. First I was interviewed and screened to see if I met the criteria for admission. I passed with flying colors, of course. After they had made the decision to take me, I had to say goodbye to my husband and I was taken to another room where they gave me some scrubs to change into. I had to change in front of them so that they could document any tattoos and scars I had and also make sure that I had nothing dangerous like razor blades on my person. They also took my things from me so that they could search them for contraband. I also had to piss in a cup, drug/alcohol test.

After all of that I was taken to a dimly lit room filled with recliner chairs and a flat screen TV. I guess this was the waiting room. There was probably around 20 or so chairs in there. It was affectionately referred to as 'The Chair Room'. I was assigned to a numbered chair and given some blankets. It was pretty late by this point so they gave me some extra meds to help me sleep and I passed out until the next morning.

2.5

When I woke up it was morning and I was so sore. The recliners looked a lot comfier than they actually were. I walked over to the nurse's station to ask if I could have a shower. They gave me some towels and a new set of scrubs, a bunch of soaps, shampoos, a toothbrush and some paste. The shower was huge, it was wonderful. It was so hot too, I never wanted to get out. When I was done I got rid of my dirty scrubs and towels and went back to my recliner. I passed the day by talking to the other patients that were sitting near me and watching the huge TV that was right in front of me. I think I was in there for a little over 24 hours.

It was the middle of the night but I was being shaken awake by a nurse. There was a bed available for me on one of the units so it was time for me to leave the chair room. It was a little bittersweet really, I was just getting comfortable, my meds were just starting to kick in. But, off I went.

The unit I was taken to wasn't that far away from the recliner room. When I got there I had a quick interview with my nurse and was then shown to my room where all of my things had been put. My roommate was already sound asleep. She was one of the girls that I had been talking to in the chair room. At least I knew I had a good roommate.

I asked my nurse for some more medication to help me get back to sleep but it was no use, I was awake now, medication wasn't going to help me get back to sleep. I lay there for what seemed like forever before the nurses came around, waking everyone up for breakfast. I was so sick of tray food by this point so I was excited to be allowed to go to the cafeteria. I hurriedly got dressed and went to join the line by the door. Before I could get out of the door they pulled me out of the line. I wasn't allowed out yet, I had to meet with the doctor and then fill out a safety plan to be approved to go to the cafeteria. I was irritated, tray food again. Yay.

Being a Saturday, I didn't get to see the Psychiatrist that I was assigned, I saw the fill in. I hated him instantly. He had me confused with other patients, he completely dismissed most of what I said to him. He did nothing to help me. He put me on medications that I told him wouldn't work. I was so furious. I wrote an enormous essay in my journal about just how much I hated him and never wanted to see him again. I told the nurses and anybody that would listen about how much I hated him. Thankfully, my assigned psychiatrist was nothing like this guy, he was fantastic.

My assigned psychiatrist listened to what I had to say. He empathized. He let me list off all of the medications I had already been through and had no luck with. He was patient while I just ranted on. He made the decision to try me on a medication that he thought would be different to the rest, one that he thought might help me. I agreed to it and started the new medication straight away.

The next day was horrible. I'm no stranger to psychotic symptoms but this caught me totally off guard. I went to the cafeteria for breakfast but had to be bought back early. The noise, it was just too much, there was so many people in there. After breakfast was group therapy. During group I was huddled in a chair, wrapped in a blanket. The noise in my head just wouldn't stop, it was so loud. Everything was loud. The voices in my head were screaming so loudly. It became unbearable and I jumped out of my seat and ran out of the room still partially wrapped up in the blanket. I burst through the doors and came to a halt right in front of the nurse's station, hyperventilating.

I was gasping for air, I was crying out, almost screaming. I was hugging myself so tightly. My Psychiatrist conveniently chose that moment to walk through the door. He saw me and instantly pulled me into his office. I could barely get out what was happening in my head. The noise.....the screaming. I sat in my chair, hugging myself, rocking back and forth. He immediately gave the order for that medication to be stopped and started me on Lithium. I also had my cafeteria privileges revoked for the rest of the day because I couldn't promise him that I could keep myself safe and not try to hurt myself. That was okay though, I didn't want to go back there, the noise....so much noise. I was allowed back to the cafeteria some time the next day. Or maybe it was the day after, I forget.

It took a few days after my meltdown before I finally started to feel better. After a few days I could be around people again and the noise in my head was almost gone, it was so much quieter in my head. My psychiatrist explained to me that when I came in I was suffering from what was called a 'Mixed Episode'. In some cases of Bipolar Disorder patients can experience episodes where they are both manic and depressed at the same time. In my case I was also experiencing psychotic symptoms, which the failed medication exacerbated. And a whole lot of anger. So much anger. But like I said, I was starting to feel better now.

2.6

While I was in hospital I went to a lot of group therapy. It looked good in my file if I went to group every day. One day during group therapy the therapist suggested that we all make lists of our symptoms to help us identify what to look out for. Some people had depression, some PTSD, others eating disorders. I have Bipolar Disorder so I made two lists. One each for Depression and Mania. Here are my lists:

<u>Mania:</u>

- Sudden impulse to get more tattoos, piercings, coloring my hair. There was one time that I messed up my hair so badly, I had to walk to the store at 3 in the morning to buy more color to dye over the 3 other colors that I just put through my hair. It was horrible.
- Making lots of plans
- Everything looks brighter, like really bright. It's beautiful
- Starting new hobbies. Oh, SO many hobbies!
- Obsessively cleaning either my whole apartment or just one particular section

- Restlessness/ unable to sit still. Literally, cannot sit still, it's exhausting
- Louder and more boisterous, confident
- Racing thoughts and pressured speech
- Wanting to do dangerous and thrilling things. Carnival rides are a favorite
- Angry/ irritable/ careless of other people's feelings
- Not sleeping or sleeping very little.
- Being able to work 12 + hour days at work on little to no sleep for days on end
- Hearing voices/ white noise/ screaming
- Visual hallucinations
- Paranoid delusions
- Interest in religion
- Spending money that I don't have
- Rash decisions

Depression:

- Trouble with sleeping
- Uncontrollable crying out of nowhere
- Anxiety
- Isolating/ not wanting to socialize with anyone
- Anger/ irritability/ careless of other people's feelings

- Thoughts of self- harm and suicide
- Cancelling plans
- Hearing voices/ white noise/ screaming
- Visual hallucinations
- Paranoid delusions

As I wrote out my lists it started to become a lot clearer to me. I am sick, I do have an illness, and that illness is Bipolar Disorder. Never before had it been so clear and obvious to me. I sat for a while to let it sink in a bit. I know that doctors had been telling me this for a while now but I was struggling to see it. Seeing it all on paper helped to change that. I could see it, bright and clear. I always knew that I was depressed and psychotic but it was the mania part that I had struggled to come to grips with.

After we were all done with our lists we made another list about things we could do to control our illnesses. Here is mine.

How To Control My Illness

- Take me medication
- Know my triggers/ avoid triggers
- Know symptoms

- Take action early. Call Psychiatrist or Psychologist
- Involve my husband more
- Understand that I have a lifelong illness. Understand that there will be good and bad days.

Taking medication, that's easy. I have an amazing app on my phone that helps me with that plus a huge medication organiser. Knowing my triggers, stress is always a huge trigger. Another trigger is breaking my routine. Having a routine helps me to have some kind of control and predictability in my life. Knowing symptoms, check. Take action, yep, I can do that. Involving my husband, I could put a bit more work into that one. Finally, understanding. I put this on the list because I feel like when I can understand and accept the illness, it will be easier to live with.

I passed the rest of my time in hospital by going to group therapy, coloring in a crap load of pictures and making a lot of bracelets in recreational therapy. My Aunt and Uncle were in the US too so they came for a visit. My medication seemed to be leveling me out a lot too so for that I was thankful. It had been a while since I felt level.

Bipolar Disorder is like a terrifying roller coaster. It just throws you around and around and around in every direction. It's a lifelong illness with terrifying lows and euphoric highs. But with medication, medication that works, it can become a little more like a child's swing, gently going back and forth. Not gone, always there. But just a little easier to handle.

Hospital V.3

The Eating Disorder

3.1

I stood on the scales, crying. I'm not entirely sure when, but sometime in the last year I gained 10 kilos and it's revolting. I used to be fit without even trying. I could eat whatever I wanted without even gaining a pound. My stomach was flat. I never even exercised. I was beautiful without any effort at all. Was.

It started about a month ago. The obsession with my weight, the dieting. It started out innocent enough. I would eat less and try to eat healthier. I walked to and from work every day. I just needed to lose 10 kilos. But it wouldn't budge. I started crying every time I looked at the scales. Which was a lot because I weighed myself probably about a hundred times a day. Unfortunately, I'm not even exaggerating, I couldn't keep off of the thing. It all spiraled out of control too fast for me to catch it. I went back and forth between bingeing and not eating anything at all.

I backed off of the scales and walked over to the toilet, grabbing my toothbrush on the way. I shoved the toothbrush down my throat and tried to make myself throw up. I don't even know why I bother though, it never works. I've long since come to the conclusion that I have no gag reflex, yet I continue to spend hours and hours, hunched over a toilet trying to make myself throw up. I sat in a heap on the floor, tears still streaming down my face, hyperventilating. I felt defective for not being able to make myself throw up. I felt worthless. I am worthless. I'm fat.

I eventually picked myself up off of the floor and went into the living room. I walked over to the couch where my bottles of pills were strewn all over the place. I had so many pills. I'm not even talking about my prescription medications either; I'm talking about diet pills, laxatives, diuretics, probiotics. I was taking more and more and more and more. The directions on my bottle of diet pills said to take two a day. I was taking 10. My psychiatrist didn't know, I hadn't told him yet. I knew that I shouldn't be taking all of these pills, I knew it but I just couldn't stop myself. I thought that my psychiatrist would be annoyed. Maybe disappointed in me. There are few things that I hate more than a psychiatrist being disappointed in me. It makes me feel like a piece of shit. I am a piece of shit.

I was miserable but I still had so much energy. After taking my handful of pills I got up and got changed. I was manic and most of my energy went towards losing weight. I was driven and determined to lose weight. I ran every single night, three miles or more. Usually more. I did sit ups and all kinds of other exercises during the day when I was at home. I became obsessed with it. I couldn't miss a day, if I did I felt horrible, I felt like a failure and I wanted to die. I was so miserable but at the same time I had all the energy in the world, all of the drive. I barely slept yet still, so much energy. I was manic but in a really bad way. It wasn't the usual brightness, happiness or good mood. It was obsessive, controlling, driven, and angry.

My eating was out of control. I would eat barely anything at all for a few days and then binge for the next few. I cried almost every time I ate because I felt so disgusting. That's a part of the reason why I was taking so many pills, I was trying to balance out my 'over eating'. I was also drinking a ridiculous amount of green tea. I drank some before every meal, before every snack. I thought that it would make the food digest and disappear quicker. I couldn't eat unless I'd had a cup of green tea. I was a mess, a disaster. It was time for hospital again and I knew it. But I didn't want to go. Until one day when I couldn't stop crying. Again with the crying.

3.2

I don't know what happened but all of a sudden I started crying again and I couldn't stop. Literally, couldn't stop. I wanted to kill myself because I couldn't get rid of the weight. I shouldn't be this fucking fat, I thought to myself. I'd always been thin before this. So I went to see the emergency doctor again. Luckily the one right by my apartment was open. I went in there, still crying and told the receptionist that I needed to see the doctor. She told me to take a seat in the waiting room. After a short while she came and got me, did my blood pressure and told me to wait in a little room for the doctor to come and see me.

The doctor seemed young so at first I was skeptical but he was fantastic. He sat with me for almost half an hour trying to figure out what was wrong with me while I sat there and just cried and cried and cried. In the end he gave me some Xanax and sent me on my way with a strict instruction to go to the hospital if I didn't feel better or if I felt worse. I laughed, can it really get that much worse? Well, it did. About a week after I saw him I went to the hospital. It had gotten worse. I was still crying, almost all day and all night. I wasn't sleeping because of the crying. I still wanted to kill myself because I was so fat. I weighed myself constantly, I was barely eating. The breaking point was when I took a razorblade to my ankle.

I got some things together, clothes, shampoo, etc and had my husband take me to the hospital. When I got there I recognized the same check in guy that was there the last time I came in. I liked him. He's pretty laid back. I checked in and waited for the first psychiatrist to come and evaluate me. They didn't have to talk to me for very long before they took me in. I told them about my dieting. All of it, the excessive exercising, all of the diet pills and laxatives etc. My obsession with my weight. I also told them that the obsession with weight was making me suicidal and that I thought I was cycling really fast between manic and depressed.

I said goodbye and hugged my husband as they took me into the chair room. It was the same deal as last time. They checked my weight, I pissed in a cup, they gave me some scrubs to put on while they checked my clothes and my person for dangerous or harmful objects. After that I was assigned to a recliner and then given some blankets and basic items like deodorant, toothbrush and paste. I didn't have to wait very long before another psychiatrist saw me.

The second psychiatrist I saw was the same guy as last time. A middle aged guy that seems like he's done this a million times. He probably has. I'm pretty sure he asked me all of the same questions as last time. He asked about my current and past diagnosis, medications, treatments. Tested my memory by having me recall some words. Again, it was all the same crap as last time.

When he was done I went to my chair and was just settling down when I got called up to the medication window to be given the new medication that the psychiatrist had just ordered for me. I took it without argument or questioning. Had I known that he had given me an antidepressant, maybe I would have refused it. Maybe not. I sure wish I had though. I did not sleep a wink that night. I was so hyper, it wasn't even funny. That whole night was just horrible. I thought that I was going to jump out of my skin. Thankfully, I only had to spend one night in the chair room. Fairly early the next morning I was moved over to my unit.

3.4

As I was being escorted over to my new unit the nurse explained to me that the hospital is under construction right now, they are building more buildings, bigger buildings, so that there will be a lot more beds. Because of that, the unit that I was sent to was partially outdoors. It was kind of cool. All of the bedrooms were enclosed, obviously, but there was a big outdoor space in the middle of it all. I liked it. It did get a little chilly at night time though.

As I waited to see my nurse I noticed that a lot of the staff on this unit were familiar to me from the last time that I was here. That was comforting. I saw my nurse and after our chat I went over to my room to unpack my things from the brown paper bags that they always put people's belongings in. After that I took a walk around the place and talked to some of the other patients there. Everyone was really nice.

At some point during the morning I saw my psychiatrist. She's the same psychiatrist that discharged me the last time that I was here. I liked her a lot, she was very friendly and listened to what I had to say. I told her everything, just like

I had with the chair room psychiatrist. When I was done she was kind enough to take me off of the horrible medication that kept me up all night last night and she gave me something for my anxiety. I slept much better after that.

Despite being able to sleep again, I didn't feel any better. I was still suicidal. I wanted to hurt myself and I was still trying to make myself throw up, even though I knew that I couldn't. I still don't know why I bothered. After a few days my nurses realized what I was doing and I was given a minder because I couldn't promise to my psychiatrist that I wouldn't hurt myself and that I wouldn't try to purge. This poor person had to follow me around absolutely everywhere that I went. Poor soul. After a couple of days though I finally decided to commit to not hurting myself or purging and my minder was reassigned elsewhere.

The day after my minder was reassigned I was in the consult room with my psychiatrist. I asked her what was wrong with me. I still wasn't really eating a great deal and I was still exercising a lot, even though I was in hospital. I couldn't run but I could do sit ups, pushups, etc. She told me that I had an eating disorder. Eating disorder Not

Otherwise Specified to be exact. She said that I couldn't be diagnosed as anorexia or bulimia because I wasn't thin enough. Wasn't thin enough. There's the joke.

I didn't know what to think. My head was spinning. I sat there, not speaking. I mean, I knew that maybe my diet wasn't okay, but to be diagnosed with an Eating Disorder? It never even occurred to me that I would have an Eating Disorder. Fuck. And it started out so innocently. It was my mania that triggered it I think. The mania caused the obsessive exercising and the obsession with food and weight. When that spiraled out of control it turned into depression and that's when it got REALLY bad. I can't remember the rest of our conversation. I zoned out. When we were done talking I got up and walked out, back to my room. I lay on my bed for a few hours trying to process our conversation.

3.5

As the days went by I did start to feel a little better. My mood had levelled out, I had stopped trying to purge, I wasn't exercising as much. Now I was just depressed and suicidal, any mania that was there was now gone. Depression isn't fun at all but at least now my mood was consistent. That's something, right? It still needed to be fixed though. I couldn't go home being depressed all of the time.

One day I was talking to one of the other patients that was on my unit. We were talking about what each other was there for. I told him about me and then he told me about how he was here having ECT, electroconvulsive therapy. At first I was shocked, I didn't know that that was still a thing. I asked him why he was having it and he said that it's because he has Bipolar disorder. He's been through so many medications and nothing ever works. I told him that I was the same, that I've been on about 30 medications by now. I was kind of curious and I asked him how he got an ECT consult. He told me he just asked his psychiatrist about it. His psychiatrist thought it could be good for him so they ordered his consult. He said that it's been really good for him and it's helping with his depression.

Over the next few days I thought about it and I thought about it. Do I really want to do something like ECT? Is it really to that point already were I don't have a whole lot of other options? 30 medications are a lot to go through. How many more are left to try? And do I really want to try them all? No. I'm tired of trying. I don't want to keep going through medications that don't even work. It's exhausting. I'm tired. I feel like a lab rat.

The next morning when I saw my psychiatrist I asked her about getting an ECT consult. I was scared, not of the ECT but of asking for a consult. I hate to ask for things, especially if it's something that my doctor hasn't already suggested. My psychiatrist though thought that it would be a great idea, that it could be a really great thing for me. She thought that I could probably get a lot of benefit from it. That maybe it could make my medications start working or even lessen how many I'm on. And so she ordered the consult and I waited. I waited two days. I thought that they were never going to come and my mood was sinking lower and lower as the hope disappeared.

It was about 6 am and my nurse was getting me out of bed. I didn't want to get up. She said that the ECT doctor was waiting to see me. As soon as she said that I opened my eyes and swung my legs out of bed. I was still half asleep though. I reached around for some clothes and then went into the bathroom to get changed out of my pajamas. A little while later I emerged from my room and went to find my nurse. She was waiting for me and directed me into the office that the doctor was waiting in.

I went in shyly and apologized for my tardiness. He turned around from his computer to look at me. He said that there was no need to apologise and asked me to sit down in the chair across from him. I instantly recognized him from my last stay here. He was the good doctor, the one that I liked. Turns out he's also the head of the ECT department.

He started bombarding me with questions about my depression, mania, psychotic symptoms. He was thorough, I'll give him that. I broke down in tears part way through his interrogation. My head was so foggy, I got so confused and tangled with all of the questions, it got too much. At the end of it though he said that I would be a very good candidate for ECT. He said that it could help me a great deal if I were willing to try it. I said that I would really like to give it a shot so he ordered an ECG, lung X-ray, and bloodwork for me. He also labelled me as high risk in my file.

3.6

Everything moved so fast. All of the tests that were ordered were done within 24 hours. I had the ECG and the lung x-ray done that day and the blood work done the next morning sometime before I even got out of bed. There's a nurse that goes around early in the morning and draws blood. You don't even have to get out of bed for it, or wake up. It's super nice.

The next day I started to have doubts about getting the ECT. I wanted it, I wanted it so bad. But what about work? What about bills? If I agreed to the ECT I would have to stay in the hospital for another month, to have the first 12 sessions. I didn't know if I could do that, I needed to go back to work to pay the bills. It stressed me out to the point where I felt physically sick. I thought that I was going to be sick. And I was shaking. Sick and shaking. I had to go back to work. I can't handle this amount of stress. So I went to find my nurse.

I found my nurse and asked her if she could pass on a message to my doctor. I didn't want the ECT. She pulled me aside and asked me if I was sure that that's what I wanted, was I sure that I wanted to turn it down. I nodded my head and said yes, I was sure. I'm a master liar. I wanted the ECT so bad but I just couldn't handle the stress of possibly not being able to pay the bills. I was also scared that I would get fired from my job. That's what anxiety does to you. It makes you turn things down, even if you want so badly to do it.

My nurse passed on the message for me and the next day I met with the doctor again. He, also, asked if I was absolutely sure that I wanted to leave, if I wanted to leave without having the ECT. He also made it clear that he thought I would be back, probably within a month. He said that medications alone were clearly not helping me, haven't been helping me, and that I wasn't a whole lot better than I was when I came into the hospital. He said that if I came back then I would be held involuntarily and they would give me the ECT. I said that's fine. He me for a little while longer, 3 days before he signed my discharge papers and I was allowed to leave.

Hospital V.4
The Electroconvulsive Therapy

4.1

Aaaannnddd, back again. In the chair room.
Motherfucker. I've already been through intake and
been assigned a recliner chair. I pulled the lever back
on my chair so that I could lay down. I don't know why
though because I couldn't stop moving. My legs
wouldn't stay still and my hands were shaking like
crazy. I felt like I was going to break out of my skin.
They gave me something, I don't know what, but it
was supposed to help me sleep and calm me down.
Well, it did the opposite. Everyone else was sleeping
but I was wide awake.

I had only been out of the hospital for one week.
Turns out the psychiatrist was right when he said that
I would be back. When I left last time though it was
mostly because of money reasons, not because I was
actually stable and ready to leave. Thanks to a brilliant
and kind hearted friend though, I was able to come
back. She started a go fund me account to raise
money for my hospital stay and ECT. I will forever be
grateful to her for what she did to help me. I don't
know what would have happened if she hadn't helped
me.

I sat up in my chair, I couldn't do this, lay down. I
needed to walk around or something. I got up out of
my chair and started to speed walk around all of the
recliner chairs. I was practically running. I didn't get
very far before one of the nurses came and stopped

me. I told them that if they wanted me to stop walking about then they would need to give me something so that I could stop moving. The nurse walked away and then came back with a little yellow pill. I took it and was passed out in my chair within half an hour.

Not long after I woke up the next morning I was taken over to a unit. It was the same one that I was on last time. They went through all of the usual crap, introduced me to my nurse, showed me my room and gave me my things. I already knew my way around the unit and there was even someone still here from my last stay. After all of that they told me that I could expect another ECT consult sometime tomorrow morning.

The next morning, I was hanging out in the day room when my nurse came and got me for my ECT consult. It was a different doctor from last time but he looked nice enough. He went through all of the same stuff that the other doctor did last time only he came to a different decision. He told me that I should continue to try more medications and that he wasn't going to recommend me for ECT. I was furious. Just two weeks ago the other doctor said that I NEEDED to have the ECT. I started to yell and cry simultaneously. He called my nurse and she gave me another one of those little yellow pills. I started to calm down shortly after. I don't know what it is about those little yellow pills, but I like them.

Later that same day, the doctor came back. He had my file from my last visit and also a copy of my first ECT consult which was done by the head of the ECT department. He told me that he had changed his mind and that I will be starting my ECT on Monday. Five days from now. I was thrilled.

Before the ECT I had to have an ECG and a lung x-ray. I'd already had those the last time I was in hospital, after my first consult. I also needed to have blood work done, which I had done the following day. Now, the big one, reducing meds. Some of my medications I can't be on while having ECT so they started tapering down three of my medications. It was scary. I'm so med sensitive that anything could happen with a med change/ decrease. But for the ECT, I was willing to do it.

The next day the doctor came to see me. He told me that they've got an ECT opening on Friday, tomorrow. This meant completely dropping those three meds that I was tapering off of. Quitting cold turkey. I was okay with that, still a little scared at what might happen but I was willing to do it because at least I was supervised. I wanted the ECT, I had so much hope for it. I thought that it was going to be some magical cure all.

4.2

It was the morning of my first ECT and I was SO hungry. I'm not allowed to eat or drink anything though. My friend said that she would smuggle me some French toast from the cafeteria for me for later. She was such a kind friend. She did this a few times for me before she got discharged. I tried to distract myself from the hunger by pacing up and down the halls for a good hour or so. Eventually I wore myself out and decided to just sit on the bench across from the nurses station and wait for someone to come and get me.

Eventually a nurse from the ECT department came to pick me up. She was very friendly looking and she had a beautiful smile. When we got to the ECT room she showed me over to my hospital bed and I got on it and lay down. She asked me if I wanted a warm blanket, I said sure. She went over to an oven looking thing and got me a blanket. It was warm, toasty warm, I'm in heaven! I called them oven blankets.

As I waited for someone to come and get me I lay there thinking. I feel like I should be scared or nervous but I'm really not. I was never afraid of having ECT. Before now it never occurred to me that I should be. Why be afraid of something that could possibly bring so much relief?

After five or ten minutes the other ECT nurse came and got me. She asked how I was doing as she wheeled my bed into the other room. I said I was fine. Always fine. In the other room the psychiatrist and the anesthesiologist were waiting for me. They both said hi. I proceeded to tell them all about the oven blankets while the anesthesiologist attempted to find a good vein in my arm, apparently I have very few. Once he found a vein he looked at me and said, 'goodnight'. I could feel the propofol go up my arm. When it reached my head, my face, it started to itch. I laughed and then passed out.

When I woke up after my first ECT I was really confused. I wasn't totally sure where I was or what was going on. This ended up happening after every ECT. I would always ask where I was and what number ECT it was. I always thought that it was my first one. When the nurses saw that I was waking up they went into the ECT room to get the psychiatrist. He rushed over to me, asking how I was feeling. I felt okay. Just a little groggy and a bit of memory loss. Also confused about why he seemed so worried. He listened to my chest and asked me a few questions. He said that my seizure had lasted for four minutes. It's only supposed to last for thirty seconds or so. Once he was sure that I was okay he said that he would add back one of my medications so that hopefully next time the seizure would be much shorter. I was unfazed. I felt fine.

4.3

I had so much energy. SO. MUCH. ENERGY. I didn't want to stop moving, couldn't stop. I was outside walking, almost running around in a little circle. I'd been doing it for some time now and I guess the nurse felt like I should stop now. My nurse came over and asked me to stop walking. I explained to her that I couldn't, I couldn't stop. I'd been walking in a circle for so long I didn't know how to stop. One of the other patients came over and told me to just try walking in the opposite direction. So I did and it worked, I fell on my ass. The other patient laughed. I immediately got up and started kicking at bushes and flowers. Then I saw a pigeon. I wanted to catch it and keep it as a pet in the draw in my room. I couldn't catch it, it was faster than me and flew away. Damn pigeon.

I don't know what I expected out of my first ECT but it definitely wasn't this. I was full blown manic. Racing thoughts, can't stop moving, can't talk coherently, manic. It was almost dinner time. I needed to burn off this energy so that I could sit down and eat in the cafeteria. I went inside and started to run up and down the hall. I just couldn't stop. I asked my nurse for one of those little yellow pills but she said that I can't have them anymore because I'm having ECT. I was pissed. Then my mood flipped. Just like that, out of nowhere, I wanted to sit in a corner and cry. But I still had so much energy. That whole night was just horrible. Truly horrible.

The next morning when I woke up I felt a bit better. All of that energy had gone, the mania was gone. Now I just felt sad again. I felt suicidal. I felt angry and irritable. I couldn't believe how manic I'd gotten the night before. I wondered if that would happen after every ECT session. I hoped not. It's too much. There once was a time when mania was enjoyable, I loved it, but not anymore. Now I think that it's just as bad, maybe worse than depression. Mania can be so destroying and devastating. The debt, the ruined relationships, the impact on work. It's not all sunshine and rainbows. The grass isn't greener.

The days between ECT sessions were usually pretty uneventful. They had a routine. First, on the night of ECT day, I would get manic. Okay, so sometimes the mania was eventful. Then I would crash and get depressed again. I was also really grumpy and irritable. I would snap at just about anyone, I didn't care who. My mood flung every which way. But there was a routine. At least it was predictable. At least I had some idea of what to expect every day.

By about my fourth ECT the doctors were starting to notice a difference in me. Before every session I had to fill out a mood disorder/ depression questionnaire. The lower the mark the better the mood. On my first ECT I scored somewhere in the forties which was just about full marks. By my fourth ECT I was down to somewhere in the twenties, which was excellent. All I'd noticed in myself was the mania/ anger/ irritability pattern after each ECT but I guess I was less depressed now too. Hip, hip, hooray. My doctor noticed something more positive though, he said that I was making a lot more eye contact and also communicating much better than what I was when I first came in. This meant a lot to me as I've always had trouble communicating and I guess when I think about it, he's right, I was improving. I was thrilled. I was finally making progress, something was finally working. I would take the mania and anger if it meant that I was less depressed. But that 'less depressed', was short lived.

4.4

I don't know what happened. I just slipped, right back into soul crushing depression. I wanted to kill myself. I wanted to die. I didn't want to be here anymore. I grabbed the extra blanket off of my bed and took it with me to the bench in front of the nurses station. I didn't want to be alone but I also didn't want to be near people so I lay down on the bench and covered myself with the blanket. I lay there for what seemed like forever and just cried. I just cried. I wanted so badly to be dead and it hurt so fucking much.

I don't know how long it took before my nurse came over to see what was going on. Long enough that the cushion I had my head on was soaked with my tears. She asked what was wrong. I said that I wanted to kill myself. Then I started ugly crying. You know the kind, when you're crying so much you start hyperventilating because you can't breathe and you have snot all over your face. I just wanted it to stop, I was so tired of hurting, I didn't want to do this anymore. My nurse got up and said that she would be back in a minute. When she came back she had some lavender hand lotion. She offered me some. I stopped crying except for a few quiet tears. The hand lotion smelt nice and it felt nice on my hands. I said thank you as I got up to go back to my room. I went to my room and had a nap until dinner time. Crying is exhausting.

I felt no better when I got up for dinner. I was also hungry though so I put on my shoes and went to join the line for the cafeteria. Dinner was good. The food there was always good. When I got back from dinner I sat in the TV room for a while and watched some meaningless crap on TV. It wasn't enough to distract me though. I still wanted to die. I decided to go and ask my nurse if I could have anything to put me to sleep, or if I could have my night meds two hours early.

My nurse said no. I wasn't allowed to have any extra meds, nor was I allowed to have my usual night meds early. I started yelling and screaming. I don't know where it came from, it just happened. It didn't get me very far. When the yelling and screaming didn't work, I stormed off to my room. In my room I had an open closet with some draws in it. I got up in my closet, on top of the draws, with my journal and started tearing up bits of paper. As I was tearing it up I was throwing it around the room. There was paper everywhere. The anger started to fade and I started laughing. I thought that it was hilarious. I was a grown ass adult throwing a temper tantrum in a hospital and throwing paper around my bedroom.

After probably five minutes of trashing my room, my nurse came to get me. She saw the mess and told me to get out of my closet. I was still laughing. She wasn't, but thankfully she wasn't angry either. I immediately

81

apologized for the mess and told her that I would clean it up. I never did, but the thought was there at least. Anyway, my nurse had gotten permission from my doctor to give me my medications early, hooray. So I took my meds and then went to bed. I didn't stay in bed for very long though before I got up again. I couldn't sleep and the meds didn't help so I spent a few hours pacing up and down the halls until one of the nurses made me go to my bedroom.

One morning, shortly after the paper tearing event, around my seventh or eighth ECT, I woke up manic. REALLY manic. All I could think about was sex. I needed sex. And this is a pretty huge deal because, except for two or three times, I don't usually crave sex when manic. It's just not a symptom that I usually have. After breakfast that morning was group therapy. At some point during group I stood up and proclaimed to the entire unit that I wanted sex, that I needed sex. Thankfully, most people just laughed at me. Later on that morning though I saw my psychiatrist and proceeded to tell him that I thought he was really hot. He didn't find it particularly funny. He took it as a cue to call my husband and have him come in for a meeting. The meeting that we apparently had I really have no recollection of. I didn't journal about it and I still have some memory loss from the ECT. That meeting is a memory lost forever I fear. Memory loss really does have its good and bad sides.

4.5

I stayed in the hospital until the day after my twelfth ECT. I'd been in there for a month. Thankfully ECT causes memory loss so it really didn't feel like I was there for that long. My psychiatrist had decided that I was stable enough to go home and I could do the rest of my treatment as an outpatient. I still had three more sessions to go for a total of fifteen. I was happy to be going home. I missed my husband and I knew that he was excited for me to be coming home. While I was in hospital his Australian visa had been approved so we were starting to plan our move. We decided to leave in about a months' time, after I was done having ECT. The plan was that I would go back to work for a couple of weeks as I would only be having the ECT once a week, that way I would still have health insurance. So, off I went, back to work. I had missed work a little, but mostly I just missed the people that I worked with.

When I went back to work, I couldn't even remember how to do my job. I'd been doing this same job for a year now, how do I just forget how to do it? All my job involved was counting and sorting money. But I couldn't do it. I lasted two days before I put in my resignation. It was really hard to have to admit that I could no longer do my job but I was useless. I totally underestimated the extent of the memory loss that I would have with the ECT, it never occurred to me that it would affect my job. Luckily I was still able to keep my health insurance for a few weeks while I finished my ECT.

As I wasn't in hospital anymore I noticed my mood swings between mania, anger, and irritability a lot more. I guess because you can get away with throwing tantrums and being a bitch a lot more in hospital than you can in the real world. As I finished up my ECT I noticed that my main mood was anger and my poor husband was the one who had to deal with it. My mood was vicious, I was vicious.

The move to Australia was turning out to be very stressful, and maybe that was having an impact on my mood. Stress usually does. We had so much stuff to still pack up and get rid of. Then there was all of our bills and the apartment, etc. In the end we ended up just deserting our apartment and also a lot of our bills. We never heard anything from the apartment owners so I guess that they figured we weren't coming back. We left a lot of our furniture and stuff in the apartment too, everything that we couldn't get rid of.

I have a lot of really amazing friends in America and it was really hard to say goodbye to a lot of them, knowing that I probably wouldn't ever be back. My husband and I had lunch with some of them and breakfast with others. They are some of the best, yet saddest memories I have of being in the US. I've never had a lot of really close friendships, I find it difficult,

I've always been like that. The friends that I have in the US though, well, they're more like family and I will always miss them.

Despite the sadness of leaving great friends, when the day finally came to leave the US my husband and I couldn't be more excited and relieved. All of the stress was worth it and the day to leave had finally come. We had stayed in a motel the night before so that we could be closer to the airport, one of our friends had dropped us off. Before we left the motel my Father in law came to spend some time and say goodbye. After that, we were off to the airport and out of the country!

Hospital V.5
The Psychotic Episode

5.1

Well, we're back in Australia. I've been away for close to five years. I haven't seen most of my family for close to five years, my parents, my siblings. I gave strict instructions for there not to be a whole bunch of people meeting us at the airport but I knew they wouldn't listen. It's not that I didn't want to see everyone it's just that I've been really emotional these past couple of weeks and I didn't want to be one of those lame ass people crying at the airport. We were walking up the ramp to the baggage collection area and I could see them all, probably about ten in all. I was so happy to see them, even though I asked for them to not all be there. My Aunt and Uncle handed me a bunch of flowers and bags full of Australian chocolate for my husband. I hugged my mother and step father, my siblings and their partners, and last of all my Grandma. I didn't know what to say to them all, it felt so surreal to be near them all again. It's been so long.

After the airport we went back to my Mum's house. We were going to stay there for a little while before moving in with my Grandma. We started unpacking all of our things and going through all of the stuff that we had already sent back with my Aunt and Uncle on their last trip. I was so overwhelmed. I was happy to be back but I still just wanted to cry. I've been like this for a couple of weeks now and I don't know why.

Everything feels so surreal and strange. I was worried that the stress of the move had triggered some kind of episode.

A few days after we got to Australia I had an appointment with my new doctor. I chose this new doctor over my old doctor because he specializes in psychiatry and that's really what I needed. I had so much stuff to tell him in a tiny ten-minute appointment. My Mum came in with me too because she wanted me to ask about disability but I was too afraid too so I asked if she could do it for me. When my name was called my Mum and I got up and followed him into his office. He was very polite and asked what I needed. I picked up my bag of medications and emptied it onto his desk. I sat in my chair hugging myself as I told him what my diagnosis was. Then I added my humongous pile of hospital records to his desk. I sat, rocking back and forth as he wrote me new prescriptions for all of my medications. When he was done he asked what else he could help me with. That's when my Mum asked about me being put on disability for a little while. He barely even thought about it before saying yes. He said that he was amazed I even worked at all this past year. He gave me a certificate for 90 days. Before I left he told me that he had put in a request for me to be assigned a case worker and a psychiatrist and labelled it as urgent. He told me to expect a call from them soon.

A few days later I got a call from my new case worker. She sounded friendly enough on the phone, she asked me to come in to meet her later that week. So I did. It was easy enough to find her, the building that she worked in was right behind the hospital. I'd never been there before, I think that it was a new building, an add on that happened while I was away. My new case worker was amazing! She put up with me as I sat there and just cried. I don't know how she even understood me as I answered her questions through floods of tears. When we were done she said that she was going to try and get me an appointment with one of the visiting psychiatrists. She said that I was labelled as urgent so it shouldn't take too long. At the very least she could get me a teleconference with one. I was scared about meeting the new psychiatrist, I always am about meeting new doctors, what if I don't like them? But I was excited because maybe she could help me. I was crying all of the time, I didn't feel like anything was real, I felt fake, I felt like I was living in my head. I'd also started to cut myself again. I was doing it on my ankle so that I could cover it over with socks and long pants. I was terrified of any one seeing it.

While I was waiting to see the psychiatrist, I saw my old doctor who I've known for about 25 years. I saw him because I wanted my tubes tied and that was one of his specialties. The thought of having children makes me feel so physically ill. I can't stand the thought of it touching me from the inside, I barely even like being touched on the outside. The whole idea of having children just makes me feel sick. It makes me want to kill myself. The doctor asked me what I would do if I were to become pregnant and I told him straight out that I would stab myself in the stomach and then jump from a building. He said that he wanted to wait a month to make sure it's really what I wanted and then he'll do it for me. I was thrilled. This was such a huge thing for me.

5.2

It didn't take long for my case worker to call me with the appointment details for my new psychiatrist and I was glad. I'd already had to see the emergency doctor once because I was going to kill myself. My appointment with the psychiatrist was about a week away. I can do this I thought, I can get through this week. I can do this. And I did, I got through the week with no more emergency doctor visits. But I was still miserable. I was crying all of the time and sometimes I didn't even really know where I was. I was living inside of my head. I had no idea what was going on. I can see it all now, in hindsight.

I waited, nervously, in the waiting room. I had no idea what this psychiatrist was going to be like. I hoped that I would like her. I jumped as my case worker called my name, I'm always off in my own little world. I followed her to a room where my psychiatrist was waiting for us. I said hello and sat down. Our conversation was lengthy but in short, this is how it went.

Me: I'm going to kill myself.
Psychiatrist: Therapy can help with that.
Me: I hurt myself.
Psychiatrist: Therapy can help with that.
Me: I've been abusing my Clonazepam.
Psychiatrist: Therapy will help with that.
Me: I want my medications changed. Today.

Psychiatrist: All of your medications are the best medications for your condition so, therapy will help.

Now, I understand that therapy does in fact help. I know that. But sometimes it takes a bit more than that. Sometimes you need to look at your medications and see if somethings not quite working. Sometimes hospital helps, sometimes you need to be on suicide watch. I don't know what I wanted her to do but I wanted her to do something, anything. I was barely holding on at that point. I was ready to find a tall building, I was ready to die. I was also very psychotic which I didn't realise at the time and I guess neither did she. Or maybe she just didn't care. The final straw though came when I told her that I was having my tubes tied. Now, as I've already mentioned being sterilized is something that I was very passionate about. She told me that I shouldn't have it done, that in ten years I would probably change my mind and regret the decision. It was at this point that I walked out. I was in tears as my case worker followed me outside. I told her that I was sorry for leaving like that but she told me that it was okay. She asked if I was going to be okay. I told her that I was going to see my doctor and that I might consider going to the hospital.

I knew that my doctor was one of the emergency doctors that day so I went straight down to the doctors clinic. For once I didn't have to wait long, there wasn't many people in the waiting room today and there were a few doctors on. I got up as my doctor called my name. I was still crying. I thought that I could hide it by wearing sunglasses but that just looked even more suspicious. I explained to him everything that happened with the psychiatrist. I don't know why, but I thought that he would be angry with me. He wasn't. He was very understanding. I told him that all I wanted was for someone to fix me, to help me. Why was that so much to ask for? Before I left his office he gave me a prescription for something to try and help calm me down. It didn't work, it made me more agitated, but at least he tried. Which is more than that horrid psychiatrist did. Maybe it was time to go back to hospital. Maybe they could help me.

5.3

I decided to give it a few days to see if I would feel any better. I didn't, and it just kept getting worse. So I made the decision to go back to hospital. That Sunday I went out with my husband, mum, and stepdad. We went out for coffee etc with plans to go to the city hospital afterwards so that I could admit myself. When we got to the hospital I was nervous, I'd never been here before. We found the emergency department okay and the guy at the counter asked for my insurance information and what I was there for. It took only a few minutes and then he asked me to take a seat and wait. I looked around, there was only a few other people in the waiting room so hopefully we wouldn't have to wait very long. We waited barely five minutes. A guy was at the door calling my name. He told me to come over and sit/ lay on the bed that he had in front of him. I felt stupid but I did as he said and he wheeled me on down to the emergency department. My family followed.

There were a lot of people in the emergency room but they moved me into a cubicle all of my own. I guess that's what they do with the psych patients. But that was okay, at least I had privacy. They told me to wait here for the on duty psychiatrist to come and see me. My family came in as a lady walked by and asked if I wanted a sandwich. I declined. I hate sandwiches. I was nervous waiting for the doctor but at least my family kept me distracted. When the doctor came I asked my family to leave the room. I don't like my family knowing how fucked up I am. The doctor asked me the usual barrage of questions which I answered truthfully, even though I was ashamed of some of my answers. I also gave them a list of medications that I've already been on and a list of every diagnosis I've ever had. I came prepared this time. At the end of our conversation he said that I would be transferred to the psychiatric hospital nearby as soon as a bed opened up. After that it was time to say goodbye to my family. I cried after they left. I felt so alone. I didn't know what to expect next.

I was in the emergency room for a long time. It could probably go down as some of the most boring hours of my life. I just sat on a hospital bed that was in a tiny yellow room painted yellow. There was also some cereal thrown on one side of the wall. Nice to know that I was in a clean hospital. After about four hours a nurse came to tell me that I was being transferred to the short stay unit as I probably wasn't going to be transferred to the other hospital until tomorrow. I was on the short stay unit for about an hour, just long enough to have dinner and half a pitcher of lemon cordial. They moved me within the hospital again, this time to the psychiatric intensive care unit (PICU for short).

The PICU wasn't very big. There were only five beds on the whole unit. The beds surrounded a tiny little room that had great big windows. That was the nurses station, it was setup so that they could see us all. In the corner, near the door, was a security guard, to make sure that none of us escaped I suppose. I guess we weren't all voluntary. There was a young girl in the bed nearest me. She looked barely more than a teenager. In the bed on the other side of me was a guy, probably about my age, who couldn't sleep. He was literally terrified of going to sleep. In one of the other beds was an older guy who walked around in a hospital gown. It wasn't very flattering, there was a lot hanging out, we'll just put it that way.

It was nearing bed time so my nurse came over to give me my medications. Usually at night time I had five pills. In the little cup there was only two. I asked where the rest of my meds were and she told me that they didn't have them all. I was pissed. But I let it go. I wasn't going to be here for long I told myself. At least I was allowed PRN's (as needed meds) if I wasn't able to sleep. And sure enough, I couldn't sleep. I was wired without all of my meds. I felt like I could bounce off of the walls. I sat up for hours, scrawling utter crap in my journal and walking around in circles. I eventually conceded defeat and asked for the valium. At least I tried. I really do hate to take sleep meds because they never work for long.

The next morning, I was woken up by cold toast and cereal. I pushed it aside and went back to sleep. I'm not a breakfast person. I eventually got up a couple of hours later. I felt gross so I asked the nurse if I could have a shower. She got me some towels and soap and things and I headed off to the units communal bathroom. At least the shower was big, I thought to myself. I turned on the shower and brushed my teeth while I waited for the water to heat up. It didn't. There was literally no hot water. I was annoyed, I was so looking forward to a nice hot shower. Oh well. I opened the bathroom door to be greeted by hospital gown guy waiting to use the toilet. I disposed of my towels and went back to my bed. It was so freaking boring there, there was nothing to do but watch the one TV that they had up on the wall. Luckily, at about 3 pm, the ambulance came to get me and take me to the psychiatric hospital nearby.

5.4

When I got to the psychiatric hospital the ambulance driver found a nurse to hand over my file to while I waited at the counter. That nurse then took me to my room to go over some paper work and go through all of my things. She was very nice. I didn't have anything restricted so I was allowed to keep all of my things. She asked me a bunch of questions and then we went back to the nurses station so she could check my blood pressure etc. After that I went back to my room to unpack my things.

I had a whole room to myself and even had my own bathroom. I couldn't wait to finally have a hot shower. It looked like a really nice hospital overall. Just as I sat down on my bed, a nurse came to get me for dinner. I was nervous and I didn't really feel like being social either. The dining room was fairly big. There were about ten round tables in there and in the wall of one end was a big window where they handed out the meals. I looked around for someone that looked nice and I asked a girl sitting by herself if I could sit with her. We both ate in silence. When I was done I disposed of my plate and went back to my room. The nurse said that a doctor would be coming to see me sometime tonight so I decided to just wait in my room until they came.

It was late when the doctor came, around 8pm, the nurses were already starting to hand out night meds.

The doctor asked me a lot of questions. I cried a lot. I told her that I was living inside of my head and I couldn't be sure who was real. I told her that it was kind of like the matrix. There was only one way to get out of my head and that was to choose between the red pill and the blue pill. The red pill would take me back to reality, the blue pill would let me die. I told her that I wasn't sure which pill I was going to take. I so badly wanted to die but I also didn't want to hurt my family again. It was a really long interview. When we were done I was exhausted and just wanted to go to bed so I hunted down my night nurse, got my meds, and went to bed.

The next morning, I was woken up by a nurse letting me know that it was almost breakfast time. When I went out to the dining room there was a few other people milling about, waiting for breakfast to be put out. I got a cup of tea and picked a table to sit at. I decided to sit by myself today. I hate feeling awkward sitting with someone and not even talking to them. Sitting by myself was much more comfortable. Every morning for breakfast I had two Weetbix with butter on them and a cup of tea. I got my meds while I was eating breakfast too. After breakfast I decided to try not to be a recluse so I sat in the common area and watched TV with a few of the other patients. Most of the people there turned out to be fairly friendly. There was just a few that kept to themselves.

Early in the afternoon I was called to come and see the doctor. It was the same doctor as last night plus a consulting psychiatrist. My nurse was there too. My nurse always sat in when I saw my doctor and/or psychiatrist. This session went much the same as last nights. A lot of crying, a lot of talking about living in my own head. A lot of telling them that I don't feel like I'm a real person. At the end of the meeting they decided to take me off of three of my medications and put me on one new one. Which was fine by me, I didn't think that some of my meds were working anyway. They took away my sleep med, anti-anxiety, and one of my mood stabilisers and added a second anti-psychotic. The anti-psychotic helped me to sleep better and, eventually, it helped me to feel like a real person again.

The first week that I was on the anti-psychotic I noticed that I was shaking a lot and my eye sight had gotten really bad. I was drinking loads and loads of water, thinking that it would help my eyesight. It didn't, but at least I was well hydrated. I still have a problem with my eye sight but the mediation works so well that I'm willing to live with it. Same with the shaking and trembling. Although that did get a little better, it's not as bad as it was when I first went on it.

5.5

This hospital stay was very boring. There wasn't a whole lot of stuff to do and a lot of people weren't really very social. After a few days though I learnt that I was allowed to leave the unit because I was there voluntarily. Sometimes I would go for a walk to the nearby grocery store and by snacks and things. Sometimes I would go for walks around the hospital grounds and nose about in all of the beautiful old buildings. A couple of times my family visited and took me out for lunch.

There was one day, at the end of the first week, when I saw the psychiatrist and I said nothing more than 'I don't know'. I find it very hard to think under pressure so usually I write a list of things to say when I see the doctors. That day though, I didn't. I didn't think that I would be seeing them that day. They asked me a lot of questions and I answered all of them with 'I don't know'. When they told me that my session was over I felt like they were angry at me, that I had made them angry. I went back to my room and cried for probably a good half an hour. When I eventually stopped crying I decided to write them a letter, apologizing for being useless. I gave it to my nurse to give to my doctor. I didn't see the doctors again for two days, you didn't get to see them every day there like you did at my last hospital. The whole time I waited to see them again I spent worrying that they hated me, that I'd made them angry. Of course, when I saw them again, they made sure to tell me that they weren't and hadn't been angry at me.

I was in the hospital for three weeks this time. The first two weeks that I was there were spent seeing how the extra anti-psychotic would work and I didn't get to see the doctors very much. I had to ambush them one day just so that I could tell them how I was doing. The antipsychotic was working well though. At the beginning of the third week talk started of possibly trying an antidepressant. Now, I've had a pretty colorful history with antidepressants, I can't take SSRI's or SNRI's at all because even with mood stabilisers and anti-psychotics, they make me manic. They decided that they wanted to try me on a low dose of an MAOI, one of the older antidepressants. If all went well, then I would get to go home soon. Antidepressants usually make me manic within a few days so we wouldn't have to wait very long to see what would happen.

I didn't know what to think of trying the antidepressant, every single other time I'd been on one I got manic or it threw me into a mixed episode. But, I was in the hospital, so I figured it was worth a shot while I was in a fairly safe environment. So I waited. I waited for the mania. And it didn't come. The first day I was on it I felt nauseous and I had the most awful headache. The second day too, I had a headache. By the third day I felt physically fine and I wasn't even manic. I was so happy. For the first time ever I was on an antidepressant and I wasn't manic. My doctors were thrilled too. They said that with the new anti-psychotic and the antidepressant, I seemed much better than I was when I first came in three weeks ago. I was no longer having hallucinations, well, only some auditory ones. I had also stopped crying all of the time and felt like a real person again. They said that it was time for me to go home. I was so excited. I was so tired of being in hospital and I really felt that, with these new medications, I would be able to stay out of hospital for a while this time. A couple of days later my husband and my mum came to pick me up and take me home.

5.6

The first few days after I got out of the hospital were a bit strange. I'd been in there for three weeks so it took me a little bit to settle in back home again. I just tried to pace myself, to not overload myself. My husband and I had been living with my mum and stepdad but always had a plan to move in with my grandma so a few days after I got out we moved. I'd lived with my grandma before so it wasn't new to me at all. My room was still basically how I left it the last time I had lived there.

The week that I got out I had a bunch of appointments. I had appointments with both of my doctors, one was to schedule my tubal ligation. Which went very well, I am thrilled to now be sterilized. I also had an appointment with my case worker. I kept really busy that week. The weeks following, I saw at least one of my doctors every week. I saw my case worker every week also and she had an appointment set up for me with the other visiting psychiatrist. She thinks that I will like this other one much better. And I did.

My new psychiatrist was kind, funny, and very to the point. No sugar coating or beating around the bush. Sometimes she swore, and I liked that. She asked me what it was that she could do for me. I said that I wasn't so sure. She went over my diagnosis to get started. She read my recent hospital notes and the ones from my other four admissions. She agreed with the notes from my last hospitalizations and diagnosed me with Bipolar I Disorder, Anxiety Disorder, and Borderline Personality Disorder. She then went over my medications with me. After that she kept going, asking me lots of questions about everything. She questioned me about how I felt, my hallucinations, how I was around other people, what school was like for me, my childhood. Everything. She was very thorough.

When she was done she stopped and looked up at me. She said that I'm obviously very smart and self-aware. That I've obviously been through a lot of crap in my life because of my illness. And then she said something that I was so obviously un prepared for. She said that I seem stable. As stable as I'm probably going to get anyway. Twelve years in the mental health system and not once has a doctor told me this. Never. I didn't know what to say. Obviously I was happy to hear this. I let out a laugh and then looked up to smile at her. I said thank you.

I was stable. Finally.

Afterward

Some parts of this book were very hard to write, I am still very emotionally raw in regards to some of it. Especially in regards to relationships and how I have sometimes hurt other people. One of the people that I hurt was my sister. We went for a good few years not speaking to each other. We started talking to each other again around the time that I was moving to the US. I love all of my family, my husband, my brother and sister, my parents. But here I would like to share with you something that my sister wrote after she read the second draft of Always Unstable.

"Growing up we lived on a farm. Our younger brother and myself would always be outside riding bikes, kicking the footy, in the shed building things, feeding the animals or just out having adventures while Megs stayed inside either playing the piano, doing crafts, reading books or just in her room on her own. She was quieter than us and kept to herself mostly. To us that just seemed normal and that's what she enjoyed doing. I mean not everyone's a tomboy like I was.

Once we were both in high school though we didn't really get along at all that much. I was the annoying little sister that she didn't want to be embarrassed by I suppose.

The first time she was hospitalised for a suicide attempt (I can't really remember how old I was, perhaps 13-14) all that I remember is that it was very rushed and we had to go stay at our Aunt and Uncles for a night or two.
I didn't really understand what was even happening to be honest. Mum eventually took us to visit her in hospital but I couldn't understand why she was even in there.
She didn't look sick?
They had an Xbox there so our brother and myself just sat in the main room and played that up until it was time to go home. Until reading Meghan's story I didn't realise that's how bad it was at the time. It just shows that because someone doesn't look sick doesn't mean they aren't. And mental illness is just as severe as a broken bone or cancer. You put as much effort into treating it as you would any other illness.

Not long after she was back home and back at school I caught her smoking behind the building with her new friends. I kept her secret and didn't tell our mum or dad because for once she was actually letting me be her friend and hang out with her.

Then the smoking turned to alcohol and drugs, but we were finally becoming closer than we had ever been and I had a sister who was also one of my best friends.

Even though I hung out with her a lot during this time she never once pressured me to follow her and she would say that she didn't want to see me go down the same path. To this day I have never taken drugs of any sort.... Except once Megs and her friends made pot cookies, I didn't know and dug into them. So really it was an accident and completely involuntary.

Over those couple of years as much as I hated seeing her abuse her body so much I was happy that I had a sister that liked me and was my friend. She actually was the first person that I came out to about being gay. She had the best reaction that I could have hoped for. She was happy and proud of me.

Pretty shortly after that though I made a decision to move 5 hours away to live with our dad to finish my schooling. I had been getting bullied at school pretty bad and was causing me to be depressed because of that. It was hard leaving everything I had ever known and my family but I knew it had to happen for me to become happy again. The first day at my new school I actually made friends and to this day they are still some of my closest, best friends. I also met the love of my life here too.

For a short stint I moved to Adelaide for maybe 8 months and during that time Megs came to stay with my roommates and myself for the weekend. That's when things changed. I won't go into detail very much but after that weekend I was left very angry, hurt and embarrassed in front of my roommates and work mates (I worked in a night club). From then onwards for the next couple years I had cut down all contact with her.

A couple years later when I had heard she was moving to America to live I thought it was probably time to repair what I could of our relationship at least back to sisters. It probably took 12 months and a few more arguments before things were okay between us again. When she started to go downhill and get hospitalised a few times it was getting quite scary for me because I was pretty much convinced that the only way I was ever going to see her again was going to be in a coffin when they bring her body home after a successful suicide attempt. I'm lucky that I work with one of my sister in-laws so that the very stressful days like when Megs was having ECT and I was at work I had her for support.

So much has happened to her in her short life so far and even after reading her story I still sometimes struggle to understand how bad it has been for her and how confusing it must be, but with what she tells us about her illness and the research I've done, I'm learning so much I didn't even know before and understanding.

I couldn't imagine going through what she does every day and I am so proud of her for getting to where she is now. She will always have my support even if she were to make me angry or hurt. I will always love her and I will always need my big sister."

I feel so blessed and fortunate to have a husband and family like mine. I got truly lucky there. I would not be here without them.

About The Author

I am 27 years old I've been living with mental illness for a very long time. But I decided long ago that I wouldn't let that define who I am anymore. I am so much more than my illnesses. I am a writer, a painter, a knitter, and an avid walker. I love the winter time; I love the rain. I also have a constantly growing collection of stuffed animals. I love tattoos.